Precision Medicine

Mbuso Mabuza

Published by Lekwandza Media, 2023.

PRECISION MEDICINE

First edition. July 7, 2023.

Copyright © 2023 Mbuso Mabuza.

ISBN: 979-8223158288

Written by Mbuso Mabuza.

Also by Mbuso Mabuza

A Healthy Mind And Best You: Achieving Great Results in Every Aspect of Your Life

Purposeful And Better You

Sustainable Development Calls for Effective Strategic Leadership for Efficient Health Systems

Health Promotion In Low Socioeconomic Settings

Medicine and Sociology of Health

Qualitative Methods In Public Health Research

Global Health Disaster Management

Global Health Policy And Programme Challenges

The Journey of Life Has a Gift of Purpose

Epidemiological Research

Ethics, Qualitative And Quantitative Methods In Public Health Research

When Love Lasts

Blockchain Technology In Healthcare

Virtual and Augmented Reality in Healthcare

Data Analytics and Healthcare Informatics

How To Improve The Way You Think

Health Systems Engineering: Building A Better Healthcare Delivery System

Artificial Intelligence In Drug Discovery And Development

Precision Medicine

Table of Contents

Preface

With the present emerging artificial intelligence (AI) technologies, computational "machine learning" techniques for training and generalisation from data, and cutting-edge statistical techniques, will play a significant role in analysing multidimensional datasets generated by the new technologies of systems medicine. This progressively but rapidly leads to a "new taxonomy," generating new approaches for disease diagnosis, therapy, and clinical decisions, promising more individualised treatments and improved outcomes for patients. Indeed, if this approach becomes efficient in clinical practice, it provides a real paradigm change in health care, from reactive to proactive medicine.

Precision medicine will allow big data patterns to emerge and algorithms to be developed, which, in turn, will allow more predictive and precise decisions about one's health to be made. Considering the rapid scientific advances in genomics and the vast adaptation of wearable technology and other quantified self-applications, it is likely only a matter of time before this data will play a larger and more integrated role in public healthcare services.

Precision medicine, sometimes called personalised medicine, is an emerging technological advancement which aims to personalise prevention and treatment according to the genetic, environmental, and lifestyle variability of individual persons or a specific group of people with commonalities, as opposed to the 'one-glove-fits-all' approach which has less consideration for the uniqueness of the individual person or specific group of people with commonalities such as similar genetic changes in a tumour. The genetic changes are determined in a special laboratory where a biopsy from the diseased organ or tissue is analysed through a process of DNA sequencing, genetic testing or molecular profiling. Once the genetic testing is completed, tailored treatment can be decided for the patient.

Perhaps, the clearest utility of precision medicine approaches thus far has emerged from efforts to improve disease diagnosis with the promise of better treatment. This perspective emerged as a critique of medical practices characterised as employing reductionist and oversimplified methods of disease categorisation.

Treatment is not the only aim of precision medicine, but prevention is also important as genetic testing for people with a family history of a certain illness such as diabetes mellitus, could also receive tailored preventive measures before those people even get sick. As such, precision or personalised medicine is driven not only by individual health data, but also by the availability of reference medical knowledge and evidence, that is, precision or personalised medicine is linking knowledge with individual health data for decision support.

Contrary to the precision medicine approach, the clinical treatment paradigm purports that a certain treatment should be given for a certain disease, such as antiretroviral therapy for people living with HIV, chemotherapy and radiation therapy for people suffering from cancer, and is oblivious of the unique genetic changes, environmental factors, lifestyle and behavioural factors of the individual and the adverse events that ensue.

The current evolution of personalised medicine is happening at a fast pace, whereby it goes beyond therapeutics selection for a patient but into the realm of drug discovery, planning and delivery of care, and engagement between consumers and companies focusing on the improvement of healthcare. Such rapid evolution of personalised medicine is largely driven by advances in diagnostics, digitalisation, data and analytics operating across a broad scope.

Nonetheless, precision or personalised medicine can be considered as the cornerstone of modern medicine. With so many hospital admissions being attributed to a 'one-size-fits-all' prescribing approach and adverse drug reactions being among the leading causes of death globally, not to mention the huge economic implications this creates, a tailored approach for every patient is needed. At the centre of this should be pharmacogenomics with the goal to improve drug safety and efficacy. Furthermore, therapy for each patient should be designed according to their personal characteristics, health status, lifestyle and pharmacogenetic profile. Ultimately, the goal of precision or personalised medicine is to contribute towards preventive, predictive and participatory health systems.

Chapter 1

Precision Medicine in the Era of Artificial Intelligence and Big Data

1.1 Introduction

With the present emerging artificial intelligence (AI) technologies, computational "machine learning" techniques for training and generalisation from data, and cutting-edge statistical techniques, will play a significant role in analysing multidimensional datasets generated by the new technologies of systems medicine. This progressively but rapidly leads to a "new taxonomy," generating new approaches for disease diagnosis, therapy, and clinical decisions, promising more individualised treatments and improved outcomes for patients. Indeed, if this approach becomes efficient in clinical practice, it provides a real paradigm change in health care, from reactive to proactive medicine.

Precision medicine (*an emerging technological advancement which aims to personalise prevention and treatment according to the genetic, environmental, and lifestyle variability of individual persons or a specific group of people with commonalities*) will allow big data patterns to emerge and algorithms to be developed, which, in turn, will allow more predictive and precise decisions about one's health to be made. Considering the rapid scientific advances in genomics and the vast adaptation of wearable technology and other quantified self-applications, it is likely only a matter of time before this data will play a larger and more integrated role in public healthcare services.

While the phrase "artificial intelligence" has become a 21st century technological buzz-term, it was first coined by scientists at a conference in Dartmouth, United States of America, in 1956 during a conference which was arranged to bring luminaries in the fields of cybernetics, mathematics, formal reasoning and other related fields of academia together, to explore problem-solving (Crighton, 2021).

Artificial Intelligence (AI) is a term used to describe a machine's ability to simulate human intelligence. It is a science and set of computational technologies that are inspired by – but typically operate quite differently from – the ways people use their nervous systems and bodies to sense, learn, reason, and take action. While the rate of progress in AI has been patchy and unpredictable, there have been significant advances since the field's inception over sixty years ago. Once a mostly academic area of study, twenty-first century AI enables a constellation of mainstream technologies that are having a substantial impact on everyday lives (Stanford University, 2016).

It is necessary to understand exactly how artificial intelligence and machine learning are individually defined. Machine learning is defined as the scientific discipline that focuses on how computers learn from data. Machine learning can be either supervised learning, which focuses on classification (e.g. sorting pictures into those with cats in and those with dogs in from a large set of images), and unsupervised learning. Unsupervised machine learning has no set outputs. The machine seeks to find patterns or groupings within unsorted data. Artificial intelligence is the broader umbrella under which machine learning lies, and which encompasses the use of technology to perform tasks that would usually require human intervention including sensing, learning, reasoning, and taking action (Bremmer, Gibbs and Mitchell, 2019).

The cumulative effects of Moore's Law mean that we now have computational power in the palm of our hand which dwarfs that used to put mankind on the moon. This immense ability to perform billions of calculations a second allows the use of decades' old mathematical tools to perform unique and highly accurate pattern recognition and analysis. In health data, this is allowing the ability to reveal associations and anomalies from previously thought random health data sets. Furthermore, the ability to create artificial neural networks (ANNs) and allow them to learn by trial and error, billions of times, creates software that evolves to solve complex problems in a nature akin to a child learning (Bremmer, Gibbs and Mitchell, 2019).

Artificial neural networks (ANNs) are the foundation of autonomous artificial intelligence. Their conceptualisation derives schematically from the functioning of the brain and neurons, in particular the encoding phase by the neural engrams, i.e. the capacity of a neural network to create memory according to the Hebbian principles. ANNs are computer algorithms that introduce numerical and statistical learning methods that themselves work through perceived stimuli and make decisions.

The simplest neural network is the perceptron. A typical neural network has an input layer, a hidden layer, and an output layer each composed of several neurons; this can go up to several thousands of neurons in each layer and up to several tenths of layer for the deepest structures. Each neuron has an input and an output, the output is a mathematical function of the input called the activation function. And each output is linked to the next neuron (input) by a connection which is weighted via a formula including a weight and a bias. The weights and biases are changed via training by back-propagation algorithm which retro-propagates the error calculated on the last layer between the expected answer and the one given by the ANN. The importance of connections between neurons increases or decreases over the training and the dataset used.

For example, the neurons in the input layer could represent the health information collected during the outpatients' clinics. The hidden layer represents the pathologies that deteriorate a specific function in an individual. And the output layer can represent the outcome of such a cluster of symptoms (on the risk for the life of the patient).

In the literature and since the last decades, we find different methods using ANN such as multi-layered perceptrons, sigmoidal multi-layer neurons, convolutional neural networks, Kohonen networks, Hopfield networks, etc.

Artificial intelligence and machine learning have excellent performance in tasks involving image interpretation, suggesting that medical specialties such as dermatology and radiology are one of the most promising applications of the technologies (Bremmer, Gibbs and Mitchell, 2019).

Patient monitoring is another application for artificial intelligence. Oxehealth, Oxford, UK, have created a medical device in Europe intended to perform spot observations of pulse and respiratory rate 'contact free' via optical and infrared sensors with no staff involvement. Its novelty means no published academic papers are available, but an unaudited case study of its use on an acute psychiatric ward showed improved in speed of observation collection and in the patient experience as they did not have to be woken to have their observations taken (Bremmer, Gibbs and Mitchell, 2019).

Some of the traditional sub-areas of AI are (Stanford University, 2016):

- Search and Planning: deal with reasoning about goal-directed behaviour Search plays a key role, for example in chess-playing programmes, in deciding which move (behaviour) will ultimately lead to a win (goal).

- Knowledge Representation and Reasoning: involves processing information (typically when in large amounts) into a structured form that can be queried more reliably and efficiently.

- Machine Learning: is a paradigm that enables systems to automatically improve their performance at a task by observing relevant data.

- Multi-Agent Systems: considers the question of how more intelligent systems interact with each other.

- Robotics: investigates fundamental aspects of sensing and acting – especially their integration – that enable a robot to behave effectively.

- Machine perception: has always played a central role in AI, partly in developing robotics, but also as a completely independent area of study.

- Social Network Analysis: investigates the effect of neighbourhood relations in influencing the behaviour of individuals and communities.

- Crowdsourcing: is yet another innovative problem-solving technique, which relies on harnessing human intelligence (typically from thousands of humans) to solve hard computational problems

⸺⊙⸺

THE ELEMENT OF AI WHICH has driven the field into the public consciousness is "deep learning". As the name suggests, deep learning networks are capable of learning, unsupervised, from data that is unstructured or unlabelled. The proviso is that they still first need to be "trained" in massive amounts of labelled data, which gives them the basis from which they can mathematically isolate and analyse patterns within subsequent huge sets of data – effectively "learning". The data input can be anything digital, from an image to a credit card purchase. The output is a response to a query – asking the machine to recognise a face in the image or verify the credit card purchase. This is the subset of AI which is helping develop technology like self-driving cars, for one, and assisting big companies to sift through mountains of data to gain insights about their customers or industries, help develop new products or deliver improved efficiencies (Crighton, 2021).

Although the separation of AI into sub-fields has enabled deep technical progress along several different fronts, synthesising intelligence at any reasonable scale invariably requires many different ideas to be integrated (Stanford University, 2016).

Artificial intelligence (AI) is unleashing the next wave of digital disruption. Global investment in AI skyrocketed to somewhere between $20 billion and $30 billion in 2016, with 90 percent of this spent on research and development and deployment, and 10 percent on AI acquisitions (Gadzala, 2018).

Gartner research suggests that AI and machine learning will eventually infiltrate just about every existing technology and analysts at the Industrial Development Corporation (IDC) predict that global investment in new intelligence technologies will exceed us$265 billion by 2023. The IDC also predicts that AI will be a key component of 90 percent of business software applications, and more than 50 percent of user interface interactions will incorporate some form of computer vision, speech recognition, natural language processing and augmented reality (Crighton, 2021).

It is projected that AI in healthcare will grow at an annualised 48 percent between 2017 and 2023. Artificial intelligence (AI) has cemented its status as a powerful technology with the ability to propel

a paradigm shift in healthcare and medicine of the 21st century and the future. The insights and values gained from AI and its subset, machine learning, are essential for predicting health outcomes and improving decision-making in healthcare and medicine. Advances in Artificial Intelligence and Machine Learning Technologies are likely to influence the way healthcare and medicine are delivered, in the sense that artificial intelligence will determine who delivers healthcare or medicine, and where and when healthcare and medicine are delivered. Ultimately, this points towards a shift away from the clinic and allows patients to access healthcare and medicine where they want, when they want it, and how they want it.

Integrating AI into the healthcare ecosystem allows for a multitude of benefits, including automating tasks and analysing big patient data sets to deliver better healthcare faster, and at a lower cost. As such, artificial intelligence presents boundless capabilities in healthcare and medicine, such as assisting clinicians to make accurate diagnostics faster and efficiently, the processing of large volumes of healthcare data or medical records much faster and efficiently in the context of healthcare service delivery, and prediction of future therapeutic drugs that could work efficiently (Phaneuf, 2021).

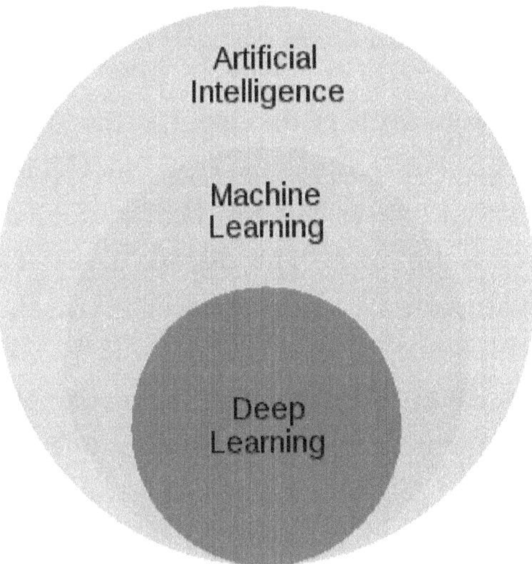

Figure 1.1 Artificial intelligence and artificial intelligence subfields as pieces put together

AI is being used or trialled for a range of healthcare and research purposes, including detection of disease, management of chronic conditions, delivery of health services, and drug discovery. AI has the potential to help address important health challenges but might be limited by the quality of available health data, and by the inability of AI to display some human characteristics (Nuffield Council on Bioethics, 2018).

The use of AI raises ethical issues, including: the potential for AI to make erroneous decisions; the question of who is responsible when AI is used to support decision-making; difficulties in validating the outputs of AI systems; inherent biases in the data used to train AI systems; ensuring the protection of potentially sensitive data; securing public trust in the development and use of AI technologies; effects on people's sense of dignity and social isolation in care situations; effects on the roles and skill-requirements of healthcare professionals; and the potential for AI to be used for malicious purposes. A key challenge will be ensuring that AI is developed and used in a way that is transparent and compatible with the public interest, whilst stimulating and driving innovation in the sector (Nuffield Council on Bioethics, 2018).

Like the web, artificial intelligence can be a positive force for political change, social change, and economic change. However, we need to ensure that all groups will also benefit from this technology. The problem today is that much of the discourse around artificial intelligence and its implications is taking place in North America and Europe (Thakur, 2018).

One tool that has been touted as a potential solution to meeting the expectations of growth or the demographic boom that is largely young and urban on the African continent is Artificial Intelligence (AI). As with many disruptive technologies, however, AI can be used for positive or negative ends. Delivering the promise of positive AI will require good systems of governance (Besaw and Filitz, 2019).

Artificial intelligence (AI) is changing society as profoundly as the steam engine and electricity have done. But unlike past technological revolutions, the AI revolution offers a unique chance to improve lives without opening up and exacerbating global inequalities. That will reduce widening of the locations where AI is done. The vast majority of experts are in North America, Europe and Asia. Africa, in particular, is barely represented. Such lack of diversity can entrench unintended algorithmic biases and build discrimination into AI products. And that is not the only gap: fewer African AI researchers and engineers means fewer opportunities to use AI to improve the lives of Africans. The research community is also missing out on talented individuals simply because they have not received the right education (Cisse, 2018).

Development and deployment of artificial intelligence in Africa is hampered by lack of connectivity, lagging technologically and other issues, but a handful of countries in the region such as Mauritius, South Africa, Seychelles, Rwanda and Senegal – spurred by the demand for economic development and recently by the need to combat COVID-19

- are laying the groundwork for innovation in the technology - making artificial intelligence a priority (Wright, 2020).

Perceptions of Africa as lagging technologically have been highlighted once again, this time by the release of the 2020 Government AI Readiness Index published by UK-based Oxford Insights. Only Mauritius, South Africa, Seychelles, Rwanda and Senegal make it into the ranking, and the report paints a gloomy picture of Africa "playing catch up in the area of artificial intelligence due to poor technological development, lack of infrastructure and a labour force that is not critical and innovative (Shearer, Stirling, Pasquarelli et al., 2020; Wright, 2020).

Africa faces several known challenges in developing AI such as a dearth of investment, paucity of specialised talent, and a lack of access to the latest global research. These hurdles are being whittled down, albeit slowly, thanks to African ingenuity and to investments by multinational companies such as IBM Research, Google, Microsoft, and Amazon, which have all opened AI labs in Africa. Innovative forms of trans-continental collaboration such as Deep Learning Indaba, which is fostering a community of AI researchers in Africa, Zindi, a platform that challenges African data scientists to solve the continent's toughest challenges, are gaining ground, buoyed by the recent "homecoming" of several globally-trained African experts in AI (Candelon, Bedraoui and Maher, 2021).

Yet, the central challenge that Africa faces in deploying AI is often overlooked: Africa's biggest companies – its national champions – are not zealously championing the cause of AI or deploying AI applications widely, causing them to trail behind global rivals. The few that have invested in AI have incurred above-average costs because they have imported talent and technology. Moreover, these companies are using AI only in limited ways. With limited bargaining power vis-à-vis foreign digital giants, and having failed so far to develop local talent, African companies run the risk of being less competitive than their multinational rivals in their home markets (Candelon, Bedraoui and Maher, 2021).

Today's company-specific AI gap will be tomorrow's national competitiveness chasm. Unless African companies actively drive the development of AI, African nations will never be able to leapfrog global rivals. Other nations have benefited from developing country-specific initiatives. Canada, Israel, and Singapore, for instance, have become globally competitive in AI by creating linkages between government, business, and academia. So can Africa (Candelon, Bedraoui and Maher, 2021).

Gender equity is critical to achieving AI fairness. Technological innovations such as artificial intelligence promise to identify and close the gender inequity gap through claims of a more data-driven, objective approach, but ironically pose another hurdle for women. Often, these digital systems inadvertently carry the same old analog gender biases (ICT Works, 2021).

There are now famous instances of the unintentional consequences of AI, such as automated resume screeners rejecting women, facial recognition disproportionately failing for women, and algorithmic credit-scores ranking women lower than men (ICT Works, 2021).

As AI tools are being tested and used in developing economies to drive insights and gain efficiencies across sectors – and as we rely more and more on them to give loans, diagnose diseases, triage medical care, and respond to humanitarian crises – we must work to prevent them from discriminating. There is an opportunity and urgency to optimise for innovative and equitable AI – especially in developing countries (ICT Works, 2021).

Development actors are taking steps to address disparities, for example, using AI to close gender-related data gaps in child marriage. Through the WomenConnect Challenge, USAID is beginning to tackle algorithmic gender bias in lending and is committed to taking action on the fair development and use of AI more broadly, working with partners to create a report and online course to better integrate AI fairness in development (ICT Works, 2021).

But we know there are many more ways that bias manifests in AI. Complex contributors to these harmful outcomes can include unrepresentative datasets, largely male data science teams, cultural norms around gender, and local policies and practices around data, among many others (ICT Works, 2021).

Responsible AI strives to be inclusive, rights-based, and sustainable in its development and implementation, ensuring that AI applications are leveraged for public benefit. Responsible AI will influence the future of information and communication technology for development.

Hearteningly for humans, Gartner's research indicates that AI and machine learning won't completely replace people because AI-driven autonomous capabilities cannot match the human brain's breadth of intelligence and dynamic general-purpose learning. Instead, they focus on well-scoped purposes, particularly for automating routine human activities (Crighton, 2021).

1.2 Expert Systems

Expert systems represent the lowest level of AI. Expert systems are comprised of a knowledge; an inference engine, which uses IF-THEN-ELSE rules to make sense of the dataset; and a user interface, where a user receives the required information. Such systems are best applied to automatic calculations and logical processes where rules and outcomes are relatively clear. 'Expert systems work the way an ideal medical student would: they take general principles about medicine and apply them to new patients" (Obermeyer and Emanuel, 2016). Despite relatively simple technology behind, expert systems could be very powerful in medical assistance. Many patient-oriented medical chatbots are based on expert systems: Florence is a practical chatbot for older patients that reminds them to take their pills (Florence – your health assistant, 2018). SafedrugBot embodies a chat messaging service that offers assistant-like support to doctors who need appropriate information about the use of drugs during breastfeeding. Efficient diagnosis assistant systems are also based on expert systems: bots like

Your.Md or CitizenDoc aim to help patients find a solution to the most common symptoms through AI. However, a chatbot never replaces an experienced doctor. If the patient's issue seems severe or doubtful, the bot itself addresses the user to an appointment with a diagnosis and eventually for the prescription of a therapy. In a specific domain concerning millions of patients with sometimes difficult access to care, some authors have described an algorithm to screen tuberculosis, based on a rule base, knowledge base, and patient database architecture. All these expert systems are based on a relatively recent subfield of computer science called machine learning.

1.3 Machine Learning Algorithms and Paradigms

Machine learning, gives "computers the ability to learn without being explicitly programmes."

As a field of study, machine learning sits at the crossroads of computer science, statistics, and a variety of other disciplines concerned with automatic improvement over time and inference and decision-making under uncertainty (Jordan and Mitchell, 2015). The uncertainty of a diagnosis inferred from a sign could be basically seen as a mathematical problem dealing with probabilities. The application of probability theory to learning from data is called Bayesian learning (Ghahramani, 2015). An algorithm is trained to execute a task (e.g., to distinguish cancer from non-cancer tissues) and to improve its performance and accuracy with experience. Depending on the amount of data and computational live judgement. Machine learning techniques often deal with a large amount of data and therefore, have a more realistic approach of biological and medical problems than "simple" mathematical science and modelization.

Three different paradigms can be classically described in machine learning. These are supervised learning, unsupervised learning, and a combined method referred to as reinforcement learning.

1.3.1 Supervised Learning

In supervised learning, the algorithm focuses on a known output; in that case the goal is to produce a probabilistic prediction y' in response to a query x'. Supervised machine learning models are trained on a pre-labelled data referred to as the training set of (x, y) pairs. The training error is roughly defined by the difference between predicted outcome y' and actual outcome y. Supervised learning systems form their predictions via a learned mapping $f(x)$, which produces an output y for each input x. Supervised learning includes several probability algorithms, like decision trees, decision forests, logistic regression, support vector machines, neural networks, kernel machines, and Bayesian classifiers (Jordan and Mitchell, 2015). The classical example in medicine is the automated interpretation of an ECG or a CT scan. These are all tasks that a trained physician can do and so the computer is often trying to approximate human performance (Deo, 2015) *and maybe surpass it*. The number of parameters of such a model is critical: more parameters reduce bias but increase noise (and random associations). The complexity of a model is a trade-off between bias and variance (Jordan and Mitchell, 2015).

The medical applications of supervised learning are diagnosis assistance for rare, difficult pathologies, and also follow-up, that needs an accurate evaluation of treatment outcome: one application on children diagnosed with cerebral palsy with support vector machines shows an overall accuracy of 96.80% in diagnosis using only two easily obtainable basic gait parameters (Kamruzzaman and Begg, 2006). Similarly, the diagnosis of valvular heart disease through neural network ensembles has been made with an accuracy of 97.4% (Das et al, 2009).

1.3.2 Unsupervised Learning

In contrast, in unsupervised learning, there are no outputs to predict. The goal is to find patterns or groupings within the data. No training is needed because there is no desired output. The underlying concept is called clustering, that is to say, the assumptions that among a dataset, the machine can automatically regroup features (symptoms, images, genes). A criterion function is defined as one that embodies these assumptions

– often making use of general statistical principles such as maximum likelihood, the method of moments, or Bayesian integration – and optimisation or sampling algorithms are developed to optimise the criterion (Jordan and Mitchell, 2015).

The "fuzzy" aspect gives the algorithm the flexibility to classify a data point to each cluster to a certain degree relating to the likelihood of belonging to that cluster. This method can detect hidden patterns across large and complex datasets. Unsupervised learning can be very useful in identifying mechanisms or risk factors for complex multifactorial diseases (Deo, 2015). Fuzzy c-means (FCM), an effective clustering method developed by Bezdek (Turing, 2018), is one of the most common instruments for medical diagnosis (Wu et al, 2015). It has already been proposed for classification of thyroid diseases (Azar and El-Said, 2013) or tumours by gene characterisation (Sun and Xu, 2014). This method also has its weaknesses: the need to determine membership cut-off, i.e., the distance from the feature to the centre of the clusters, roughly represented by the mean of the considered data and the fact that clusters are formed whatever the inputs, i.e., if the data belong to no cluster at all, the algorithm will do it anyway, thus potentially leading to errors. FCM has shown its efficiency in primary headache, where diagnosis is often difficult. The algorithm showed an accuracy (proportion of true results – whether positive or negative) of 0.97 for migraine (Wu et al, 2015).

1.3.3 A Combined Method: Reinforcement Learning

Instead of training examples that indicate the correct output for a given input, the training data in reinforcement learning are assumed to provide only an indication as to whether an action is correct or not. The action taken by the algorithm is reinforced by a reward if it is correct; if the action is incorrect, the problem of finding the correct one remains.

1.4 DEEP LEARNING

Unsupervised learning and reinforcement learning are the fundamental principles for deep learning that are applied among successive layers of the dataset. Dee learning discovers intricate structure in large datasets by using the back-propagation algorithm to indicate how a machine should change its internal parameters that are used to compute the representation in each layer from the representation in the previous layer (LeCun et al, 2015). Deep learning can therefore offer an exciting solution to incomplete biomedical knowledge: these methods can discover new biomarkers without any human input, conceivably generating truly unexpected discoveries (Oakden-Rayner et al, 2017).

Some algorithm results have demonstrated similar performance to human experts in the assessment of diabetic retinopathy, dermatological lesions (Esteva et al, 2017), atrial fibrillation screening (Halcox et al, 2017), or Parkinson's disease (Ma et al, 2014).

1.4 ALGORITHMS FOR Decision-Making

Medical knowledge and publications are increasing exponentially. As explicitly describe by Mesko: "in 1950, it was estimated that the doubling time for medical knowledge was about 50 years. In 1980 it was about 7 years for medical knowledge to double. In 2010, it only took about 3.5 years. It was estimated that by the year 2020, it would take only 73 days for the volume of medical knowledge to double". In the domain of physician trained in epidemiology, it would take an estimated 627.5 hours per month to evaluate 23 million articles on PubMed (Alper et al, 2004). The quantity of medical knowledge is simply impossible for a person to retain even if this person was reading the material all day long, whereas a computer program can read all the data, store the relevant information, and use it to help in medical decision-making. These kinds of algorithms are based on the natural language processing (NLP); they can understand a text written by a person and extract intent, sentiment, or meaning.

The IBM AI program, Watson, launched its special algorithm for oncologists able to provide clinicians evidence-based treatment options. The purpose is to support tumour board meetings: "Watson for Oncology has an advanced ability to analyse the meaning and context of structured and unstructured data in clinical notes and reports that may be critical to selecting a treatment pathway, combining attributes from the patient's file with clinical expertise, external research, and literature data" (Mesko, 2017).

1.5 Algorithms in Radiology: The Era of Radiomics

Traditionally, medical imaging has been a subjective or qualitative science. Nowadays, the amount of imaging datasets combined to computational methods provides a comprehensive quantification combined to visual assessment (Larue et al, 2017). The use of computational algorithms to analyse medical images is now called "radiomics" (Oakden-Rayner et al, 2017; Kumar et al, 2012; Lambin et al, 2012). Even if the authors may not all agree with the extent of this new domain, a large definition of radiomics can include two machine learning-applied procedures: classical image analysis with human eyes-defined features which is derived from supervised learning and deep learning with feature learning, whose principle is close to an unsupervised learning (Oakden-Rayner et al, 2017).

Response evaluation criteria in solid tumours (RECIST) is a set of published rules that define cancer evolution during treatments, and was originally published in February 2000. Nowadays, the many clinical trials evaluating cancer treatments for objective response in solid tumours are using the RECIST platform, which is developed by Parexel Informatics. This kind of standardised criteria, still dependent on the physician's observation, can be considered as the first step to replace the radiologist's eye by the computer. In magnetic resonance imaging (MRI), some research in prostate cancer has shown that textural features were significantly correlated with Gleason score (Gnep et al, 2017; Wibmer et al, 2015).

In supervised radiomics, the methodology can be resumed in four steps: image acquisition, extracting radiomics features from the images, training the computer and validating a prognosis score. The extracting stage still needs human experts' intervention as image features still are human-defined features.

These "image features" are mathematical descriptions of the visual properties of an image, describing the low-level visual information present in an image, such as the intensity / brightness and the texture of image regions (Kumar et al, 2012; Lambin et al, 2012).

A radiomic biomarker definition requires robust approaches that analyse all of the available variations in an image. Deep learning appears to be an ideal tool to accomplish this goal.

Chapter 2
The Impact of Precision Medicine

2.1 Introduction

The reductionist approach of biological organisation, with the help of traditional mathematics and physics, has successfully identified many of the components and many of the interactions but, unfortunately, offers no convincing concepts or methods to understand how system properties emerge. Information technology (IT) offers the ability to treat and organise large amounts of data and leads to a paradigm of integration – in opposition to reduction – to explain biological systems and phenomenon (Andre, 2019). Quantitative datasets of DNA, RNA, proteins, and metabolites provide an unprecedented starting point to understand the effects of perturbations on a cell (Sauer et al, 2007) and, with addition of clinical tests and imaging, the effect on the whole body. The informational view of biology defines biological information – biomarker – as a given data integrated in a network. This leads to a "systems" approach to physiology and pathophysiology. It means changing our philosophy, in the full sense of the term (Noble, 1960).

Systems biology is then a holistic approach to deciphering the complexity of biological systems that starts from the understanding that the networks, which form the whole of living organisms, are more than the sum of their parts (so-called reductionism). It is collaborative, integrating many scientific disciplines – biology, computer science, engineering, bioinformatics, physics, and others – to predict how these systems change over time and under varying conditions (ISBUSA, 2018).

With the present emerging artificial intelligence (AI) technologies, computational "machine learning" techniques for training and generalisation from data, and cutting-edge statistical techniques, will play a significant role in analysing multidimensional datasets generated by the new technologies of systems medicine (Schadt et al, 2010). This progressively but rapidly leads to a "new taxonomy," generating new approaches for disease diagnosis, therapy, and clinical decisions, promising more individualised treatments and improved outcomes for patients (National Research Council Committee on AFfDaNToD, 2011). Indeed, if this approach becomes efficient in clinical practice, it provides a real paradigm change in health care, from reactive to proactive medicine. This proactive approach is already promising in "long-term" management of diseases: chronic illnesses (Sagner et al, 2017), infectious diseases (Bengoechea, 2012), or cancer (Tian, 2012).

The concept of "4P" medicine, that is predictive, preventive, personalised, and participatory, has been advocated since more than a decade now (Andre, 2019).

Actually, the 4P medicine concept has emerged from the convergence of three trends (Flores et al, 2013):

- The increasing ability of systems biology and systems medicine to decipher the biological complexity of disease: Each pathology is seen as a personal experience and a dynamic network which is dysregulated from health to disease, and conversely, treatment is a pathway from disease to health, considering each personal dimension from molecular to social and its participation in the pathological state.
- The increasing ability of computers to integrate, store, analyse, and communicate data from medical records, symptoms, clinical tests, biological samples, imaging, and molecular biology: Then, a personalised data cloud can be imagined, including multiple dimensions of each individual, from genetic

to phenotypic characteristics, but also sociometrics (social, education, familial context, etc.).
- The increasing access to information for patients and consequently their interest in managing their own health. The digital tools not only connect recent science fundamental discoveries to clinical applications but also the patients and health-care consumers. There is an increasing phenomenon for people to go online to investigate a medical condition (Fox and Duggan, 2013).

Drug research could also benefit from these tools. Indeed, the omics data analysis would not only allow the identification of new biomarkers representative of pathologies but also propose new therapeutic targets for the development of more effective drugs (Andre, 2019).

Precision Medicine, sometimes called personalised medicine, is an emerging technological advancement which aims to personalise prevention and treatment according to the genetic, environmental, and lifestyle variability of individual persons or a specific group of people with commonalities, as opposed to the one-glove-fits-all approach which has less consideration for the uniqueness of the individual person or specific group of people with commonalities such as similar genetic changes in a tumour. The genetic changes are determined in a special laboratory where a biopsy from the diseased organ or tissue is analysed through a process of DNA sequencing, genetic testing or molecular profiling. Once the genetic testing is completed, tailored treatment can be decided for the patient.

Perhaps, the clearest utility of precision medicine approaches thus far has emerged from efforts to improve disease diagnosis with the promise of better treatment. This perspective emerged as a critique of medical practices characterised as employing reductionist and oversimplified methods of disease categorisation (Ramaswami, Bayer and Galea, 2018).

Treatment is not the only aim of precision medicine, but prevention is also important as genetic testing for people with a family history of a certain illness such as diabetes mellitus, could also receive tailored preventive measures before those people even get sick. As such, precision or personalised medicine is driven not only by individual health data, but also by the availability of reference medical knowledge and evidence, that is, precision or personalised medicine is linking knowledge with individual health data for decision support (Kalda et al, 2015).

As such, precision medicine debunks the one-glove-fits all or clinical treatment paradigm which is a trial and error approach wherein all individuals presenting with some constellation of symptoms receive a similar treatment. Contrary to the precision medicine approach, the clinical treatment paradigm purports that a certain treatment should be given for a certain disease, such as antiretroviral therapy for people living with HIV, chemotherapy and radiation therapy for people suffering from cancer, and is oblivious of the unique genetic changes, environmental factors, lifestyle and behavioural factors of the individual and the adverse events that ensue.

Although personalised medicine has been there even during Hippocrates' time, where the emphasis was on giving the right medicine, to the right person, and at the right time; historically, the concept of modern day personalised medicine was first mentioned in a monograph title in 1998. While some of the field's core concepts date back to the early 1960s, the basic idea can be credited to the Canadian physician, Sir William Osler (1849-1919) who recognised that no two individuals react or behave alike under the abnormal conditions we know as disease (Primorac et al, 2020).

The current evolution of personalised medicine is happening at a fast pace, whereby it goes beyond therapeutics selection for a patient but into the realm of drug discovery, planning and delivery of care, and engagement between consumers and companies focusing on the improvement of healthcare. Such rapid evolution of personalised medicine is largely driven by advances in diagnostics, digitalisation, data and analytics operating across a broad scope.

In recent times, the explosive growth of precision or personalised medicine has ceased to be just a basic science but it has incorporated -omics such as the correlations of protein expressions and specific diseases at cellular level (proteomics), how the molecular composition of certain genes are responsible for the production of certain proteins (genomics), and how certain metabolic processes at cellular level are associated with the expression of certain diseases (metabolomics). Ultimately, in precision medicine, the aim of understanding genomics, proteomics and metabolomics is to customise medical practice with a focus on the individual, based on the use of genetic tests, identification of biomarkers, and development of precisely targeted individualised drug treatments (Iriart, 2019).

Precision medicine then seeks to incorporate technology into medicine to create a data ecosystem that can better identify, treat, an individual patient's disease. This approach aims to seamlessly integrate clinical phenotypes and biological information, from imaging to laboratory tests (including –omics data) and health records. The rationale is to develop a new taxonomy of human disease based on molecular biology (Ramaswami, Bayer and Galea, 2018).

Over the past decade, precision medicine approaches have received significant investment to create new therapies, learn more about disease processes, and potentially prevent diseases before they arise. However, in many ways, precision medicine investments may come at the expense of existing public health measures that could have a greater impact on population health. As we tackle burgeoning public health concerns, such as obesity, and chronic diseases, such as cancer, and diabetes, among others, it is not clear whether precision medicine is aligned with public health or in conflict with its goals (Ramaswami, Bayer and Galea, 2018).

Nonetheless, precision or personalised medicine can be considered as the cornerstone of modern medicine. With so many hospital admissions being attributed to a 'one-size-fits-all' prescribing approach and adverse drug reactions being among the leading causes of death globally, not to mention the huge economic implications this creates, a tailored approach for every patient is needed. At the centre of this should be pharmacogenomics with the goal to improve drug safety and efficacy. Furthermore, therapy for each patient should be designed according to their personal characteristics, health status, lifestyle and pharmacogenetic profile. Ultimately, the goal of precision or personalised medicine is to contribute towards preventive, predictive and participatory health systems (Primorac et al, 2020; Kalda et al, 2015).

Disease Diagnostics, Prognostics, Prediction and Classification models can be used to estimate the probability of either having a particular disease (diagnostic model) or developing a particular disease (prognostic model).

In clinical practice these models are used to inform care providers and patients about decision-making regarding the disease and guide therapeutic management (Hendriksen et al, 2013).

The widespread use of prostate specific antigen (PSA) for early detection led to improved survival but at the cost of over-diagnosis, often associated with over-treatment and its adverse events. Over-diagnosis and difficulties in prognosticating clinical outcome among patients with similar histological and clinical parameters often lead to over- or under-treatment. There is thus an unmet need for new markers to sustainably improve the diagnosis and risk assessment, thereby providing a more accurate treatment decision for each individual patient (Bronimann et al, 2020).

In the challenging field of chronic fibrosing ILDs with a progressive phenotype, successful biomarker development should improve the diagnosis and prediction of longitudinal disease behaviour (such as, identifying the subgroups of patients most at risk of disease progression), as well as monitoring and enabling measurement of the outcomes of treatment. In the future, it is hoped that the ongoing implementation of multiple biomarker analyses in large international, prospective, and adequately powered clinical studies will deliver clinically significant data that will convince physicians of the value of using biomarkers at multiple stages of the diagnosis and management of chronic fibrosing interstitial lung diseases with a progressive phenotype (Inoue et al, 2020).

Predicting diseases such as heart disease is a complex task since it requires experience along with advanced knowledge. Internet of Things (IoT) technology has lately been adopted in healthcare systems to collect sensor values for heart disease diagnosis and prediction. Many researchers have focused on the diagnosis of heart disease, yet the accuracy of the diagnosis results is low. To address this issue, an IoT framework is proposed to evaluate heart disease more accurately using a Modified Deep Convolutional Neural Network (MDCNN). The smart watch and heart monitor device that is attached to the patient monitors the blood pressure and electrocardiogram (ECG). The MDCNN is utilised for classifying the received sensor data into normal and abnormal. The performance of the system is analysed by comparing the proposed MDCNN with existing deep learning neural networks and logistic regression. The results demonstrate that the proposed MDCNN based heart disease prediction system performs better than other methods. The proposed method shows that for the maximum number of records, the MDCNN achieves an accuracy of 98.2 percent which is better than existing classifiers (Khan, 2020).

Classification methods vary, and they can be used individually or in combination to analyse patient-related data sets and to create inferences for diagnosis and prediction of diseases. As such, it is crucial that an appropriate classification method be used for meaningful diagnosis and prediction of diseases (Jha et al, 2018).

According to Gog et al (2020), early identification of COVID-19 patients at risk of progression to severe disease will lead to better management and optimal use of medical resources. The prediction and prognostic risk normogram they had constructed could identify and predict COVID-19 patients at risk of severe disease, and Red Cell Distribution Width (RDW) was also valuable for this prediction. The normogram was especially valuable for risk stratification management, which would be helpful for alleviating insufficiency of medical resources and reducing mortality.

Wynants et al (2021) argue that several diagnostic and prognostic models for COVID-19 are currently available and they all report moderate to excellent discrimination. However, these models are all at high risk of bias, mainly because of model overfitting, inappropriate model evaluation (e.g. calibration ignored), use of inappropriate data sources and unclear reporting. Therefore, their performance estimates are probably optimistic and not representative for the target population. Sharing data and expertise for the validation and updating of COVID-19 related prediction models is urgently needed.

The use of a chi-square with principal component analysis (PCA) was the most consistent and preferable method to improve the prediction of machine learning models. The goal for the classifier was to predict whether a patient has heart disease. Use of features is not feasible when the system resources need to be considered. Dimensionality reduction techniques were successfully applied to improve the raw data results. The method can be applied to many real-life applications or in other medical diagnoses to analyse great amounts of data and identify the risk factors involved in different diseases (Garate-Escamila, El Hassani and Andres, 2020).

The arrival of **clinical genomics** has heralded a new era in health care. Genomic testing, involving the examination of a person's DNA, can provide information on patient susceptibility to some diseases or abnormalities and even inform how someone may respond to different intervention types, including both physical and pharmaceutical interventions. Clinical genomics tests are becoming more affordable, more relevant, and more widely used, with the number of tests performed in routine health care expected to rise at an exponential rate. Owing to its increasing prevalence and visibility in clinical care, clinical genomics has a growing importance for patient assessment and management in variety of settings, including primary care, hospital settings, and physical therapist management (Cornwall et al, 2018).

Clinical genomics involves the utilisation of one of several methods to extract and examine genetic material from human cells. These methods extract DNA from cell nuclei, allowing sequences of DNA to be compared to known databases that include information on disease likelihood, phenotype prevalence, or drug efficacy. Such investigations include molecular tests to identify variations in single gens that may lead to genetic disorders, chromosomal genetic tests to identify large genetic changes that can cause different conditions, and biochemical tests to study the amount or activity level of various proteins that may indicate changes to the DNA, resulting in a predisposition to certain disorders. Examples of such testing include tests for cystic fibrosis or for identifying risk of developing breast cancer. Emerging evidence also suggests that genetic testing may help to identify risk for persistent musculoskeletal pain following traumatic injury (Cornwall et al, 2018)

Perhaps, unsurprisingly, many medical schools worldwide have recognised the need for education in genomic medicine and are planning accordingly, whereas other health care professions are already embracing clinical genomics. The rapid expansion of clinical genomics is not unique to clinical medicine or nursing practice, nor is it restricted to a laboratory-based research environment. The advancement of clinical genomics has witnessed explosive growth in the number of at-home genetic tests now widely available through direct-to-consumer services such as those provided by 23andMe (Cornwall et al, 2018).

Clinical genomics represents a paradigm shifting change to health service delivery and practice across many conditions and life-stages. Introducing this complex technology into an already complex health system is a significant challenge that cannot be managed in a reductionist way. To build robust and sustainable, high quality delivery systems we need to step back and view the interconnected landscape of policymakers, funders, managers, multidisciplinary teams of clinicians, patients and families, and health care, research, education, and philanthropic institutions as a dynamic whole (Long, 2021).

Clinical Genomics is related to precision or personalised medicine as it enables clinicians to make diagnosis and treatment decisions for an individual or a group of people with similar genetic mutations. Clinical genomics focuses on detecting and analysing the composition of genes at molecular level to enable clinicians to characterise the cause of illness, more rapidly, less expensively, and more precisely than traditional techniques such as immunoblotting. Clinical genomics employs novel detection techniques such as DNA microarrays to genotype defective or mutation areas of a genome. Other novel detection techniques include nanopore sequencing which entails observing electrical current changes as the DNA passes through a nanometre scale, or enzymatic cleavage of the DNA base pairs to identify mutations or defects at molecular level of genes.

2.2 Biomarkers in Precision Medicine

Since the advent of genomics, the suffix "-omics" has been added to the names of many fields to refer to large-scale studies to identify biomarkers. The –omics data analysis would not only allow the identification of new biomarkers representative of pathologies but also propose new therapeutic targets for the development of more effective drugs (Andre, 2019).

Identifying effective biomarkers for prognosis and diagnosis has been considered as one of the greatest challenges in recent years. It allows for cross-disciplinary medicine between biomedical knowledge and the clinic. However, the complexity of the diseases and their heterogeneity make the discovery and valuation of efficient biomarkers very difficult. To make the interpretation of biomarkers useful and applicable in a clinical context, it is necessary to ensure the reliability of the methods employed from their detection until their diffusion. The identification of new biomarkers goes through different stages (Markman, 2013).

- Discovery
- Qualification
- Verification
- Optimisation of clinical trials
- Clinical validation
- Diffusion

2.3 Genomics

The computer methods developed in genetic research have made it possible to build a large database trying to gather and map all the discoveries in the field of DNA-protein interactions. Broad-spectrum chromatin immunoprecipitation (ChIP) (Johnson et al, 2007) methods associated with high-throughput sequencing (HTP) technologies have thus been identified and currently constitute databases frequently used in genomic research or any other type of research known as "omics" (since the advent of genomics, the suffix "omics" has been added to many field names for large-scale or genome-wide studies).

2.4 Proteomics

Protein is the product of gene expression: by its derivatives, it represents the functional aspect and dynamics of the cell. Studying the variations in the amount of a protein from its synthesis to its function makes it possible to deduce cellular homeostasis with great precision. The proteomic level, combined with the metabolomics level, is a very dynamic parameter. It is therefore interesting to study protein biomarkers representative of various cellular activities (Piterri and Hanash, 2010) and their dysfunction, for example, neuromuscular degeneration in Duchenne's disease (Hthout et al, 2016).

The screening and management of cancers also benefit from proteomic biomarker research, particularly by the early administration of drug adjuvants in locally advanced cancers in a personalised manner

(Pellegrini et al, 2011). Indeed, the cancerous manifestations are closely related to the synthesis pathways of inflammatory proteins called cytokines.

It seems that the analysis of the synthesis rate o peptide segments by new sequencing technologies is a tool for the future in transversal medicine and to unite bioinformatics with clinical practice. To date, experimental methods, aiming to associate bioinformatics with medical research, have identified 254 protein translation abnormalities (Huang and Zhu, 2017; Tu et al, 2014), resulting from an anomaly in the spatial configuration of proteins) likely to be involved in pathologic manifestations. Twenty-five protein syntheses have been identified as biomarker potential in the specific recognition of diseases.

Therefore, proteomics (exhaustive analysis of the battery of proteins expressed by a given tissue or cell population and its variations according to the physiological or pathological state) is in full expansion: it has become accessible to many laboratories, in particular through the development and modernisation of mass sprectrometry. In association with studies in genomics and metabolomics, it presents a link of the future between bioinformatics and clinical practice: whether in the identification of biomarkers in the real-time analysis of the evolution of diseases or in the evaluation of drug treatment.

2.5 MicroRNA Biomarkers (Transcriptomics)

In addition to proteomic research previously described, recognition of microRNAs (miRNAs) as potential biomarkers is intensifying. The new sequencing methods (RNA sequencing or RNA-Seq) allowed a very precise exploration of the RNA sequences and to map the transcriptome complex. The latter is a reflection of cellular activity. It allows to discover many non-coding RNA sequences such as miRNA (microRNA), siRNA (short interfering RNA), piRNA (piwi-interacting RNA), and IncRNA (long non-coding RNA) involved in epigenetic mechanisms. These RNA sequences are known to be nono-coding and intervene in the regulation of gene expression at transcriptional and post-transcriptional stages.

Non-coding RNA sequences such as miRNAs, siRNAs, and piRNAs seem to play a specific role in the compaction state of DNA, especially in the formation of heterochromatin, which is possible, thanks to histone proteins, but also in the methylation of DNA strands and the inhibition of genetic sequence called silencing. Long RNA sequences (>200 nucleotides) can also influence gene expression at specific genome locations. The study of miRNAs has specifically led to a better understanding of the genetic mechanisms underlying diabetes or cancers (Pescador et al, 2013). In addition to the different biomarker potentials previously mentioned, databases are now dedicated to the study of miRNAs.

A good application is the diagnosis of musculoskeletal pathologies. In 2013, the discovery of microRNA linked to the dystrophin protein made it possible to understand the evolution of Duchenne muscular dystrophy (Roberts et al, 2013). miRNAs are excellent biomarkers for the physio-pathological analysis of musculoskeletal tissue, and they allow the identification of many pathologies.

2.6 Biomarkers of Circadian Rhythms

Other biomarkers are particularly useful in physiopathology, in particular to identify their evolution over time. These include molecules whose quantity changes with the rhythm of biological cycles such as the circadian rhythm. Most of the endogenous biological variations are due to the circadian rhythm which makes it possible to ensure the control, the synthesis, the renewal, and the degradation of the basic molecules necessary for cellular mechanisms.

Molecules evolving at the rate of the biological clock can identify upstream pathophysiological phenomena, such as breast cancer or psychiatric disorders. These molecules are intimately related to hormonal mechanisms (Rattan, 2018).

2.7 Biomarkers of Inflammation

In recent years, a strong link between the microbiota, the digestive tract, and the brain has been highlighted. This link is undoubtedly a major avenue of exploration in biomedical research in the years to come (Sherwin et al, 2016).

This underlies endocrine, autonomic, immunological, and metabolic mechanisms. This combination of physiologies makes it possible to protect the nourishing pathways of the body by chemical feedback to ensure the body's internal homeostasis is in the external environment (Sandhu et al, 2017). New studies have identified biomarkers of low back pain. Low back pain is the leading cause of disability, caused by a variety of spinal disorders, including intervertebral disc degeneration, disc herniation, spinal stenosis, and facet arthritis. The discovery of these biomarkers is crucial in understanding everyday pain.

Since precision medicine has a new disease taxonomy of classifying disease by mechanism and molecular diagnosis, instead of looking at organs and symptoms like the mechanistic doctor's sick care, it is proposed that precision medicine will enable more accuracy in healthcare and medicine, targeting interventions to the individual, maximising benefits and minimising harm (Twilt, 2016; McLellan, 2014). Such paradigm will rely heavily on the narrative and knowledge that precision medicine will not only benefit individuals but will lead to transformative improvements in population health, what has been termed precision public health, and will optimise disease prevention strategies (Ginsburg and Phillips, 2018).

Disease diagnostics, prognostics, predictive and classification are ***user-friendly, scalable, reliable, expandable, can enhance accuracy and would assist healthcare professionals in better decision-making*** (Jha et al, 2018). There is a challenge, though, because of high dimensionality of human organ databases such as the heart database which makes diagnostics prognostics, prediction and classification difficult (Jha et al, 2018). In addition to embedding the disease diagnostics, prognostics, predictive and classification models into the healthcare professionals' workflow, there is a need for making healthcare professionals acquainted with these models for better adoption of this technology in healthcare and medicine (Jain and Singh, 2018; Kappen et al, 2016).

When genomic sequencing is used to address a specific clinical condition both the ***provider and patient*** have a say in terms of whether to screen for secondary findings or results that are not directly linked to the primary motivation for testing (Brothers, Vassy and Green, 2019).

RNA sequencing is a promising candidate for clinical applications. Studies on differential gene expression analysis have shown that increasing biological replicates improve the accuracy of gene quantifications. The advantages to using DNA methylation analysis for clinical profiling are: the analysis does not rely on the genetic alterations of the diseases; thus, it can be applied to diseases with sparse somatic mutations; the material under analysis is DNA, which is advantageous because DNA is less sensitive to heat or enzymatic degradation than RNA, resulting in more accurate profiling (Vijay et al, 2016).

In terms of clinical utility, ***clinical utility*** is difficult to quantify in genomics, in large part because the current and potential usage of genomics in medicine is so varied. In clinical genetics, clinical utility's definition ranges from definitively informing medical management to produce a positive health outcome, to satisfying the need for patients and their families to have a diagnosis, regardless the outcome. As such, the use of genomics in medicine will exacerbate this issue because genomics brings with it a social narrative of exaggerated determinism. It is also a field of medical science that is changing with particular rapidity and one in which providers feel particularly underprepared (Delaney et al, 2016).

There is lack of evidence to understand variant pathogenicity and penetrance in diverse populations, as well as impacts of disclosure on individuals, families, healthcare professionals, and on healthcare systems (Ormonroyd et al, 2018).

One of the biggest challenges in going from bench to bedside in genome sequencing studies is the accurate and reproducible analysis of the resulting terabytes of data (Vijay et al, 2016). If both genomics and clinical investigation are complex in isolation, combining them multiplies the challenge. The fact that genomic studies of human population require larger sample sizes requiring many investigators and coordination across multiple institutions with all logical challenges is particularly problematic in unbiased genome-wide studies (Altshuler and Altshuler, 2004). Currently, genetic testing is used far more frequently to answer specific clinical questions than they are to screen healthy individuals for conditions they have not yet developed (Brothers, Vassy and Green, 2019).

Regarding population screening in the public health context, local efforts are focused on maximising access and uptake rather than careful consideration of individual risks and benefits. The reality is that it is not yet known whether the benefits of genomic screening in the general population will outweigh its potential harms (Brothers, Vassy and Green, 2019).

Like other medical interventions, clinical tests – whether diagnostic or preventive – involve some *risk of harm*. The most conspicuous harms from clinical tests are false-positive results, which may lead to actions or procedures that may cause unintended morbidity and mortality. The risk for false-positive results is particularly high in genomic testing. The extremely large number of sites interrogated with exome or genome sequencing increases the statistical likelihood that one or more analytical false-positive results will be generated (Brothers, Vassy and Green, 2019).

But even if all variant calls are confirmed by an orthogonal technology as some have recommended, genomic variants may be interpreted inaccurately, or they may be interpreted accurately but the disease condition may never manifest. Rare or novel genomic variants occur commonly in human genomes and may initially be classified as pathogenic only to later be proven benign. Newer large-scale population-based sequencing data are demonstrating that the penetrance of many common pathogenic variants is lower than initially estimated. In practice, then, many pathogenic variants will be returned to individuals who will never develop the medical condition (Brothers, Vassy and Green, 2019).

False-negative results are also relatively common in genomic tests and raise important concerns. Many genes contributing to risk for specific conditions have not yet been identified, and the pathogenicity of many variants within gees that are clearly associated with disease is often uncertain. In addition, current analytical pipelines can miss pathogenic variants because of structural variation or changes in regulatory regions (Brothers, Vassy and Green, 2019).

These potential blind spots contribute to a well-known challenge in clinical genetics: false reassurance. There is a dramatic difference between telling a patient they are not at risk for a condition and telling them no genetic factors that increase their risk were identified, but the distinction between these messages may be muddled by providers or misunderstood by patients. As a result, patients can be left believing that they are not at increased risk for a condition or even that they are entirely free of risk for that condition. This false reassurance may cause patients to forego other types of screening that would normally be recommended, including mammograms and colonoscopies. If this happens, they might have been better off having never had a genomic screen (Brothers, Vassy and Green, 2019).

These factors remind us that genomic tests are far less deterministic than is generally believed and therefore not exceptional, but that they reflect the common clinical and public health challenge of balancing medical harms with medical benefits (Brothers, Vassy and Green, 2019).

While it has its own challenges, clinical genomics presents a number of opportunities in healthcare and medicine. With ever decreasing sequencing cost and increasing detection of possible drug targets, exomeseq covering larger areas of the genome has the potential for wider application in *clinical diagnosis and prognostic decisions*. DNA methylation provides a complementary approach to clinical measures for patient classification. There are opportunities for leveraging electronic health records data. The fact that many aspects of patient care increasingly incorporate genomics and informatics has implications of a transition to electronic health records for clinical genomics, including genetic testing. There are opportunities for genomics and chronic illnesses. Genomics approaches are important for preventing and managing chronic illnesses such as diabetes and inflammatory bowel disease (Vijay et al, 2016).

Personalised healthcare and ***direct-to-consumer*** genomics is another opportunity for clinical genomics in healthcare and medicine. Statistical models can incorporate genomic features and family history, coupled with factors such as age, weight, and ethnicity, for disease risk prediction in healthy individuals. People are empowered by the implementation of direct-to-consumer tools which make information including classical Mendelian diseases and prediction of predispositions to complex diseases and drug response contained in the genetic testing registry accessible to interested individuals. Federal policies in the United States of America are changing to reflect the shift to clinical genomics (Vijay et al, 2016).

With novel technological developments in single-cell sequencing, subpopulations can now be measured directly and at a previously unprecedented resolution. Single-cell sequencing will add a new level to clinical applications of tumour sequencing by increasing the resolution with which we can model complex dynamics and incorporate that into prognosis assessment and drug efficacy prediction. This suggests that single-cell resolution is necessary to accurately characterise complex tissue samples.

There are opportunities for better infrastructure, support for IRB approvals, ease of submission, and ease of access. An added benefit is that all these sequencing data are submitted to curated repositories with publication such as the database of Genotypes and Phenotypes, the

Sequencing Reads Archive, and the Gene Expression Omnibus. This publicly available data will help alleviate the issue of small sample sizes common in clinical settings and/or rare diseases. There are also pipelines with guided user interfaces that facilitate these steps, such as STORMseq, Genesifter, Ingenuity variant analysis software, and more (Vijay et al, 2016).

Advances in Genomics Approaches for Neurobiology with large-scale efforts in mapping the human brain using cutting edge brain imaging techniques, high volume data approaches are becoming increasingly useful. This enables understanding mutations and predispositions especially to Alzheimer's and autism spectrum disorders would allow for early intervention, which is often the only hope for therapy (Vijay et al, 2016).

National and international personalised medicine initiatives and Federal changes in clinical genomics in the United States of America and the success of the IMPACT and IMPACT2 studies occurring on a global scale, are inspiring international cooperation to advance medicine (Vijay et al, 2016).

In the context of provider-ordered preventive testing in healthy adults, the current state of evidence provides an opportunity to explore the potential for genomic screening to improve preventive care in healthy persons. This will determine if this technology really does carry utility as a screening test (Brothers, Vassy and Green, 2019).

Given the current state of evidence, translational research studies provide a useful opportunity for interested institutions and providers to explore the potential for genomic screening to improve preventive care in healthy persons. Offering screening in a hybrid clinical/research setting, such as the MedSeq Project, provides the opportunity to engage patients in an appropriate informed consent process. Perhaps, most importantly, this approach, in conjunction with trans-institutional efforts like the National Institutes of Health – funded Clinical Sequencing and Exploratory Research consortium, will provide the opportunity to develop the evidence base to establish whether this technology really does carry utility as a screening test. Experience on other domains of screening has led to the development of effective practices that can be used to maximise benefits and minimise risks when performing genomic testing (Brothers, Vassy and Green, 2019).

While genomic data is voluminous, it lacks variety, velocity, and veracity compared to other fields. The number of analysts working with a given dataset is small, as is the number of transactions on any given genome. The data are neither fused with other data types nor networked with other cases. The time frame for integrating clinical genome sequencing into clinical practice cannot be predicted on scientific development; rather integration depends on concerted efforts among and between the healthcare stakeholders in precision medicine (Delaney et al, 2016).

Precision medicine has been branded about as an emerging new route towards yielding substantial healthcare *cost* savings (Ginsburg and Phillips, 2018). However, the question remains, as to whether or not precision medicine will be available and accessible to all including those below the poverty line, mainly in developing countries, or it will serve the interests of big corporations interested in making a fortune in the market.

The market for disease diagnostics, prognostics, predictive and classification is likely to grow due to aging population especially in developed countries. While there are cost savings to countries due to reduced disease incidence rates as a result of implementing effective and efficient disease diagnostics, prognostics, predictive and classification models, the actual process of implementing disease diagnostics, prognostics, predictive, and classification models can be costly, more so, for developing countries.

The high cost of the instruments for single-molecule sequencing has limited the adoption of clinical genomics technology in healthcare and medicine. It is an opportunity that sequencing has promising clinical utility. The lower cost of sequencing has made sequencing more accessible to the medical community for diagnostic support (Vijay et al, 2016). However, the global economic crisis is a threat to growth of the clinical genomics market.

Many ***providers and patients*** are still sceptical about precision medicine as it is growing at a frenetic pace and yet no clear awareness about this technology is conducted. While it cannot be refuted that precision medicine as a new paradigm in healthcare and medicine could have benefits for individuals and populations, it is also critical to put more emphasis on understanding the human needs and the overall experience of patients within the healthcare ecosystem (McLellan, 2014). All key stakeholders especially providers and consumers must be involved in the planning and implementation of precision medicine for it to achieve its full potential, and this will require a multipronged approach from a socio-cultural, scientific, religious, clinical, economic and policy agenda.

Lack of or poor adoption of disease diagnostics, prognostics, prediction and prognostics may be due to lack of acceptance by healthcare professionals. Healthcare professionals may view this technology as a burden and sometimes as something that will result in them losing their jobs. The threat to society in the context of disease diagnostics, prognostics, prediction and classification is the increasing age of population and growth in the burden of disease in both developing and developed countries. The need for education and more transparency is key to address the low confidence among both providers and consumers in the healthcare and medicine ecosystem.

In some cases, healthcare providers are not rapidly incorporating clinical genomic sequencing into their practice of medicine because they are unaware, many lack self-confidence about their own knowledge and skills for using them. Many providers are also concerned about the high cost of genomic tests, the lack of reimbursement, and scepticism about the validity and utility of the tests currently being offered (Delaney et al, 2016).

There is lack of wide engagement and education with the public and healthcare professionals about understanding the application of clinical genomics in healthcare and medicine in both developing and developed countries (Ormonroyd et al, 2018).

Regarding reimbursement decisions for new technologies, newer technologies such as genetic testing may be reimbursed inconsistently or not at all. Today, genomic testing in the non-oncological space is inconsistently covered throughout the United States of America, which makes it extremely complicated for clinicians to apply such testing in the clinical arena. It is difficult to predict how this may be resolved, as payers seem to be asking for evidence from clinical utility studies that will take considerable time to accrue (Delaney et al, 2016).

The lack of *regulations* or a policy agenda while the field of precision medicine is changing so rapidly creates challenges for providers and consumers. Protecting individuals and populations against big corporations is key as excessive attention on technological innovations such as precision medicine diverts focus from the importance of ethical healthcare and medical practice. As such, clear regulations or a policy agenda must be put in place to enable wider adoption or integration of precision medicine into healthcare and medicine, bearing in mind that the public should be cautious of all overrated promises of technological innovations such as precision medicine as these could be industry marketing tools and aimed at serving vested interests.

Regulations are being developed or have been implemented in some countries and regions in order to address the issue of disease diagnostics, prognostics, prediction and classification. However, other countries and regions have not even started planning to put in place any regulation or policy in that regard. Where regulations or policies are being planned or already implemented, it is proposed that organisations or institutions that do not comply with standards will be fined. As such, there is need to focus on education and quality standards for both manufactures, providers and consumers in the healthcare and medicine ecosystem.

When the planned or implanted regulations in certain countries and regions, it is worrying that there is ambiguous liability as there is no case law or no indication of who will be liable if things go wrong with disease diagnostics, prognostics, prediction and classification. Even if there were to be globally applicable regulations for disease diagnostics, prognostics, prediction and classification in healthcare and medicine, such regulations would fall short because it is not possible to rationalise as different countries or regions require different formulas.

Research involving human subjects poses a unique set of challenges, largely attributable to the complexity of the human population, the need to respect patient autonomy, and pressure on highly distributed systems of clinical care. The demands of informed consent and data protection compete with financial pressures that have left clinicians barely enough time for patient care, let alone research (Altshuler and Altshuler, 2004).

In the realm of genomics, FDA plans for oversight are widely regarded as flawed because the FDA may lack statutory authority to regulate laboratory-developed tests

(LDTs), has an antiquated and unwieldly medical device framework that is not well aligned with the rapidly changing technical and evidence base in genomics, and may inhibit discovery and innovation – in the absence of evidence of harm – by insisting upon pre-market review of both analytical and clinical validity (Delaney et al, 2016).

The local jurisdiction of review boards and the lack of universal information technologies for managing patient information make it difficult to compare data across institutions even after regulations have been met (Altshuler and Altshuler, 2004).

Even if there were to be globally applicable regulations for clinical genomics in healthcare and medicine, such regulations would fall short because it is not possible to rationalise as different countries or regions require different formulas.

"In Canada, the rapid development of sophisticated biomarkers is disrupting the prevention, diagnosis, and treatment of illness – indeed, defining existing diseases and their prognoses. Canada has pockets of strength in precision medicine, and a nascent research strategy has been led by CIHR. However, what is notably absent is a national strategy for innovation. That is, implementing these concepts into front-line care. It is particularly important to develop and begin following a roadmap to ensure that Canada's healthcare information and communications technology will support these data-intensive models of care and the rapid-cycle innovations that characterise precision medicine as a field. The Advisory Panel for Healthcare Innovation in Canada urged the scaling-up of models of care in subfields of precision medicine that are relatively more mature, such as pharmacogenomics and cancer diagnosis and treatment. It is perceived that there is substantial potential for the commercialisation of made-in Canada concepts and tools in the precision medicine field, provided that a nimble implementation strategy can be launched as recommended" (Ministry of Health - Canada, 2015)

"To fully realise the integration of precision medicine into medicine, a policy agenda must be implemented. The growth of precision medicine brings both opportunities and challenges. There continues to be a need for high quality evidence that precision medicine actually improves outcomes if it is to be widely adopted. The policy challenge is how to obtain the needed evidence when the field is growing and changing so rapidly that the gold standard of large randomised clinical trials may be infeasible. The implementation of precision medicine will require access to large-scale, detailed, and highly integrated patient data.

Given that new health care innovations typically take years to be adopted, it is not surprising that the integration of precision medicine into clinical care has been slower than some observers have predicted. As with all new health care interventions, implementation will be stymied if such interventions do not provide demonstrated value or payers and consumers are unwilling to pay for them. Patients and consumers must be participants in precision medicine for it to achieve its potential.

One focus of future work should be the increasing emphasis on the ability of precision medicine to impact not only individuals but also populations – what has been termed "precision public health". The full realisation of precision medicine's disruptive potential will require a multipronged scientific, clinical and policy agenda. The precision medicine ecosystem's stakeholders – participants, patients, providers, payers and regulators each will require evidence of value in terms of quality of life, quality of medical care and efficiency and effectiveness optimised for cost. If successful, more care will occur before disease is apparent – a shift from disease treatment to disease prevention and early detection" (Ginsburg and Phillips, 2018).

"Individual-centred attempts to change health behaviours are ineffective. Advocates of precision medicine claim that advances and implementation of new technologies will optimise prevention strategies. However, regardless of how technologically sophisticated a society may evolve, citizens should be very careful with all these promises because: an excessive emphasis in technological solutions to prevent or treat disease diverts our attention from the root of the problem, bearing in mind that health relies on favourable social circumstances; in addition, clinical medicine and precision prevention have become an industry advertisement tool.

Protecting individuals against big corporations in the current political scenario may sound naïve given the constant economic inequalities experienced in the world in the last decades. In a fair world, healthy living directly threatens many powerful corporations.

Overrated precision medicine promises may be serving vested interests, by dictating priorities in the research agenda and justifying the exorbitant healthcare expenditure in our finance-based medicine. If societies aspire to address strong risk factors for non-communicable diseases, they will require downplaying the numerous promises of precision medicine and a greater appreciation of the importance of spending more resources on the foundational conditions that shape the health of the populations" (Rey-Lopez, De Sa and De Rezebde, 2018).

"In the next coming years many genomic discovery platforms in combination with clinical phenotyping based on electronic medical record data will lead to more insight with respect to disease processes and lead to more individualised targeted treatment. Overall, the use of clinical phenotype and classification tools help to diagnose disease early to allow a more rapid introduction of targeted treatment avoiding harm and increasing benefit" (Twilt, 2016).

"It is urgent that European bodies which have the capacity to stimulate development of knowledge through centralised platforms which ensure high quality of qualification and validation of biomarkers get their acts together if we want to make precision medicine a given rather than a fortuitous happening, generating false hope for the patients and the scientific community. Access to patients for clinical research needs new set-ups for raid identification of patients by sub-groups in a pre-competitive manner for rapid assignment according to target, treatment, and/or trials in the best interest of the patient. Patients need to be informed about the latest scientific advances, and Europe also needs a new set-up to ensure high-quality biomarker identification to allow secured treatment access.

New solutions are needed for optimal benchmarking of emerging technologies across and within classes of agents. The concept one drug, one target, one protocol; is no longer the way forward. Key questions anticipating the real-life implementation of new drugs need to be addressed early on. Long-term toxicity monitoring of mechanism-based therapies needs a new set-up beyond registration of drugs and into real-life for prolonged time. Clinical research data sets representing a selection of the population provide robust and systematic longitudinal access to data for learning which must then be confirmed in real-life settings. There is no integrated European solution to optimally learn, across cohorts of patients, patterns of resistance and relapse as patients receive treatments and/or enter clinical trials during the evolution of their disease.

This is a major limiting factor in addressing one of the key oncology challenges known as tumour heterogeneity. Integrated solution would be key in addressing regulatory endpoints linked to the current scenario by which the evolution of the disease driven by clonal heterogeneity selection is at stake. Independent data capture for all types of clinical, biological, and imaging data records alongside biomarker test results and all therapies received, in databases which are constantly curated and annotated, would be critical for benchmarking and validating new clinical trial methodology, as well as benchmarking clinical situations when randomisation may not be possible.

Solutions taking the continuum of drug development for optimal access to the forefront clinical trials but that would also enable benchmarking clinical research and real-life could be integrated into new processes, where applied comparative effectiveness research supports the decisions taken by Health Technology Assessment bodies and payers, rather than often too artificially designed registration trials. A major transformation of clinical research building on the strengths and complementarity of stakeholders working alongside new business models must be tackled" (Lacombe, Meunier and Golfinopoulos, 2017).

"Precision medicine will allow big data patterns to emerge and algorithms to be developed, which, in turn, will allow more predictive and precise decisions about one's health to be made. Considering the rapid scientific advances in genomics and the vast adaptation of wearable technology and other quantifies self-applications, it is likely only a matter of time before this data will play a larger and more integrated role in public healthcare services. This article aims at presenting a vision of how genomic and quantified data might be integrated into the Swedish public healthcare system.

Medicine needs to become more multi-disciplinary, and, in the future, there might be a new kind of medical specialisation emerging, with a focus on informatics and genomics. This means that the way medical staff is taught and how they practise medicine needs to change as well. How might we create a system that encourages patient participation?

Challenges to implementation of precision medicine in Scandinavia include the issue of buy-in from healthcare practitioners and would need to be supported by the country's administrators; and training of doctors, health coaches and healthcare practitioners needs to include more knowledge about genomics and behavioural sciences, and this may require longer years of training before these professional will join the workforce" (McLellan, 2014).

"In terms of clinical utility, clinical utility is difficult to quantify in genomics, in large part because the current and potential usage of genomics in medicine is so varied. In clinical genetics, clinical utility's definition ranges from definitively informing medical management to produce a positive health outcome, to satisfying the need for patients and their families to have a diagnosis, regardless the outcome. As such, the use of genomics in medicine will exacerbate this issue because genomics brings with it a social narrative of exaggerated determinism. It is also a field of medical science that is changing with particular rapidity and one in which providers feel particularly underprepared.

Regulation challenges are evident in the context of clinical genomics. Much as the U.S. Food and Drug Administration (FDA) is regarded as the body to regulate access to medical technologies, in the realm of genomics, FDA plans for oversight are widely regarded as flawed because the FDA may lack statutory authority to regulate laboratory-developed tests

(LDTs), has an antiquated and unwieldly medical device framework that is not well aligned with the rapidly changing technical and evidence base in genomics, and may inhibit discovery and innovation – in the absence of evidence of harm – by insisting upon pre-market review of both analytical and clinical validity.

Regarding reimbursement decisions for new technologies, newer technologies such as genetic testing may be reimbursed inconsistently or not at all. Today, genomic testing in the non-oncological space is inconsistently covered throughout the United States of America, which makes it extremely complicated for clinicians to apply such testing in the clinical arena. It is difficult to predict how this may be resolved, as payers seem to be asking for evidence from clinical utility studies that will take considerable time to accrue.

Data management and scalability challenges reflect missing standards, lack of modern data science, and inconsistent security practices, all of which prevent industrial-grade solutions. While genomic data is voluminous, it lacks variety, velocity, and veracity compared to other fields. The number of analysis working with a given dataset is small, as is the number of transactions on any given genome. The data are neither fused with other data types nor networked with other cases.

Questions may be asked as to why healthcare providers are not rapidly incorporating clinical genomic sequencing into their practice of medicine. In some cases, it is because they are unaware, many lack self-confidence about their own knowledge and skills for using them. Many providers are also concerned about the high cost of genomic tests, the lack of reimbursement, and scepticism about the validity and utility of the tests currently being offered.

The time frame for integrating clinical genome sequencing into clinical practice cannot be predicted on scientific development; rather integration depends on concerted efforts among and between the healthcare stakeholders in precision medicine. Providers, payers, and patients along with policy makers and regulators, industry and academia share the expertise and interest to push toward clinical care powered in part by genetics and genomics" (Delaney et al, 2016).

"Research findings show that healthcare professionals and researchers engaged in genomic medicine in Oxford believe that present policy around secondary findings should be considered conditional; evidence is required to understand variant pathogenicity and penetrance in diverse populations, as well as impacts of disclosure on individuals, families, healthcare professionals, and on healthcare systems. While evidence accumulates, we advocate for a cautious, limited approach, and urge wide engagement and education with the public and healthcare professionals" (Ormonroyd et al, 2018).

"Computational analysis of multi-omics data is a challenge. One of the biggest challenges in going from bench to bedside in sequencing studies is the accurate and reproducible analysis of the resulting terabytes of data.

Single-molecule sequencing is a challenge. The high cost of the instruments for single-molecule sequencing has limited the adoption of such technology in healthcare and medicine.

It is an opportunity that sequencing has promising clinical utility. The lower cost of sequencing has made sequencing more accessible to the medical community for diagnostic support.

There are opportunities for DNA sequencing for clinical applications. With ever decreasing sequencing cost and increasing detection of possible drug targets, exomeseq covering larger areas of the genome has the potential for wider application in clinical diagnosis and prognostic decisions.

RNA sequencing is a promising candidate for clinical applications. Studies on differential gene expression analysis have shown that increasing biological replicates improve the accuracy of gene quantifications.

It is an opportunity that DNA methylation provides a complementary approach to clinical measures for patient classification. The advantages to using DNA methylation analysis for clinical profiling are: the analysis does not rely on the genetic alterations of the diseases;

thus, it can be applied to diseases with sparse somatic mutations; the material under analysis is DNA, which is advantageous because DNA is less sensitive to heat or enzymatic degradation than RNA, resulting in more accurate profiling.

There are opportunities for leveraging electronic health records data. The fact that many aspects of patient care increasingly incorporate genomics and informatics has implications of a transition to electronic health records for clinical genomics, including genetic testing.

There are opportunities for genomics and chronic illnesses. Genomics approaches are important for preventing and managing chronic illnesses such as diabetes and inflammatory bowel disease.

The opportunities for personalised healthcare and direct-to-consumer genomics. Statistical models can incorporate genomic features and family history, coupled with factors such as age, weight, and ethnicity, for disease risk prediction in healthy individuals. People are empowered by the implementation of direct-to-consumer tools which make information including classical Mendelian diseases and prediction of predispositions to complex diseases and drug response contained in the genetic testing registry accessible to interested individuals. Federal policies in the United States of America are changing to reflect the shift to clinical genomics.

There are opportunities for genomics and cancer. With novel technological developments in single-cell sequencing, we can now measure subpopulations directly and at a previously unprecedented resolution. Single-cell sequencing will add a new level to clinical applications of tumour sequencing by increasing the resolution with which we can model complex dynamics and incorporate that into prognosis assessment and drug efficacy prediction. This suggests that single-cell resolution is necessary to accurately characterise complex tissue samples. There are opportunities for better infrastructure, support for IRB approvals, ease of submission, and ease of access. An added benefit is that all these sequencing data are submitted to curated repositories with publication such as the database of Genotypes and Phenotypes, the Sequencing Reads Archive, and the Gene Expression Omnibus. This publicly available data will help alleviate the issue of small sample sizes common in clinical settings and/or rare diseases. There are also pipelines with guided user interfaces that facilitate these steps, such as STORMseq, Genesifter, Ingenuity variant analysis software, and more.

There are opportunities in Genomics Approaches for Neurobiology. Advances in Genomics Approaches for Neurobiology with large-scale efforts in mapping the human brain using cutting edge brain imaging techniques, high volume data approaches are becoming increasingly useful. This enables understanding mutations and predispositions especially to Alzheimer's and autism spectrum disorders would allow for early intervention, which is often the only hope for therapy.

There are opportunities for National and international personalised medicine initiatives. National and international personalised medicine initiatives and Federal changes in clinical genomics in the United States of America and the success of the IMPACT and IMPACT2 studies occurring on a global scale, are inspiring international cooperation to advance medicine" (Vijay et al, 2016).

"Research involving human subjects poses a unique set of challenges, largely attributable to the complexity of the human population, the need to respect patient autonomy, and pressure on highly distributed systems of clinical care. The demands of informed consent and data protection compete with financial pressures that have left clinicians barely enough time for patient care, let alone research.

The local jurisdiction of review boards and the lack of universal information technologies for managing patient information make it difficult to compare data across institutions even after regulations have been met. If both genomics and clinical investigation are complex in isolation, combining them multiplies the challenge. The fact that genomic studies of human population require larger sample sizes requiring many investigators and coordination across multiple institutions with all logical challenges is particularly problematic in unbiased genome-wide studies" (Altshuler and Altshuler, 2004).

Clinical genomics presents organisational implications. Most biomedical research is well served by the traditional model of individual laboratories led by a single principal investigator, but clinical genomics research often requires multiple investigators and focused attention on the importance of teamwork in biomedical science (Altshuler and Altshuler, 2004).

There are implications for institutional change. Allowing sustained, multidisciplinary teamwork to become a viable and attractive option for biomedical research demands cultural and structural change – change that will only be brought about by academic institutions and the faculty who work in them" (Altshuler and Altshuler, 2004).

In their study, Brothers, Vassy and Green (2019) highlight that "there are benefits and challenges of indication-driven clinical testing and opportunistic screening. Currently, genetic testing is used far more frequently to answer specific clinical questions than they are to screen healthy individuals for conditions they have not yet developed. When genomic sequencing is used to address a specific clinical condition both the provider and patient have a say in terms of whether to screen for secondary findings or results that are not directly linked to the primary motivation for testing.

In the context of provider-ordered preventive testing in healthy adults, the current state of evidence provides an opportunity to explore the potential for genomic screening to improve preventive care in healthy persons. This will determine if this technology really does carry utility as a screening test.

Regarding population screening in the public health context, local efforts are focused on maximising access and uptake rather than careful consideration of individual risks and benefits. The reality is that it is not yet known whether the benefits of genomic screening in the general population will outweigh its potential harms. Until there is evidence, regulatory bodies should continue to encourage restraint in the application of genomic screens in the public health setting, and funding agencies should continue to support research that rigorously evaluates the risks and benefits of this new technology across multiple clinical and public health contexts.

Despite superficial similarities, there are important and fundamental differences in the way medical risks and benefits can be addressed in the context of provider-ordered predispositional testing in healthy adults, indication-based testing with opportunistic screening of secondary results, and population screening in the public health context. Recommendations to report secondary genomic findings should not be interpreted as an endorsement of population genomic screening. Ongoing work is developing the evidence that will be needed to fully justify current future initiative in population genomic screening. Ongoing work is developing the evidence that will be needed to fully justify current and future initiatives in population genomic screening."

Despite the great promise of big data and omics interpretation, many experts admit that these computational tools will not be sufficient to meet the challenge of deciphering biological complexity. Domain expertise in biology is essential, where decades of research can be leveraged to help interpret this data. As Philippi and Kohler (2006) say, "Without a deep and growing understanding of biological phenomena and networks, it will not be possible to find the critical signals in the tremendous noise generated by vast heterogeneous data" (Kohler et al, 2006). Moreover, this ubiquitous definition of self for every human being could lead to an "overmedicalisation" effect, with potential harms of excessive preventive measure (Vogt et al, 2016).

To fully realise the integration of precision medicine into medicine, a policy agenda must be implemented. The growth of precision medicine brings both opportunities and challenges. There continues to be a need for high quality evidence that precision medicine actually improves outcomes if it is to be widely adopted. The policy challenge is how to obtain the needed evidence when the field is growing and changing so rapidly that the gold standard of large randomised clinical trials may be infeasible. Given that new health care innovations typically take years to be adopted, it is not surprising that the integration of precision medicine into clinical care has been slower than some observers have predicted. As with all new health care interventions, implementation will be stymied if such interventions do not provide demonstrated value or payers and consumers are unwilling to pay for them. Patients and consumers must be participants in precision medicine for it to achieve its potential (Ginsburg and Phillips, 2018).

Challenges to implementation of precision medicine in both developing and developed countries include the issue of buy-in from healthcare practitioners and would need to be supported by the country's administrators; and training of doctors, health coaches and healthcare practitioners' needs to include more knowledge about genomics and behavioural sciences, and this may require longer years of training before these professional will join the workforce (McLellan, 2014).

Clinical genomics presents organisational implications. Most biomedical research is well served by the traditional model of individual laboratories led by a single principal investigator, but clinical genomics research often requires multiple investigators and focused attention on the importance of teamwork in biomedical science (Altshuler and Altshuler, 2004).

There are implications for institutional change. Allowing sustained, multidisciplinary teamwork to become a viable and attractive option for biomedical research demands cultural and structural change – change that will only be brought about by academic institutions and the faculty who work in them (Altshuler and Altshuler, 2004).

Despite superficial similarities, there are important and fundamental differences in the way medical risks and benefits can be addressed in the context of provider-ordered predispositional testing in healthy adults, indication-based testing with opportunistic screening of secondary results, and population screening in the public health context. Recommendations to report secondary genomic findings should not be interpreted as an endorsement of population genomic screening. Ongoing work is developing the evidence that will be needed to fully justify current and future initiatives in population genomic screening (Brothers, Vassy and Green, 2019).

Until there is evidence, regulatory bodies should continue to encourage restraint in the application of genomic screens in the public health setting, and funding agencies should continue to support research that rigorously evaluates the risks and benefits of this new technology across multiple clinical and public health contexts (Brothers, Vassy and Green, 2019).

Chapter 3
Future Perspectives

Artificial intelligence, combined with uniquely human capabilities, will deliver more than just efficiency – it will add value and drive business growth. This combination of machine learning and human ingenuity can be referred to as 'applied intelligence'. It will revolutionise how customers interact with businesses and how citizens interact with governments. As artificial intelligence matures, it can propel economic growth and serve as a powerful remedy for stagnant productivity and labour shortages. However, artificial intelligence will demand new skills, the redefinition of jobs and recalibration of business culture and leadership (Accenture, 2019).

Precision medicine will allow big data patterns to emerge and algorithms to be developed, which, in turn, will allow more predictive and precise decisions about one's health to be made. Considering the rapid scientific advances in genomics and the vast adaptation of wearable technology and other quantifies self-applications, it is likely only a matter of time before this data will play a larger and more integrated role in public healthcare services (McLellan, 2014).

One focus of future work should be the increasing emphasis on the ability of precision medicine to impact not only individuals but also populations – what has been termed "precision public health". The full realisation of precision medicine's disruptive potential will require a multipronged scientific, clinical and policy agenda. The precision medicine ecosystem's stakeholders – participants, patients, providers, payers and regulators each will require evidence of value in terms of quality of life, quality of medical care and efficiency and effectiveness optimised for cost. If successful, more care will occur before disease is apparent – a shift from disease treatment to disease prevention and early detection (Ginsburg and Phillips, 2018).

Individual-centred attempts to change health behaviours are ineffective. Advocates of precision medicine claim that advances and implementation of new technologies will optimise prevention strategies. However, regardless of how technologically sophisticated a society may evolve, citizens should be very careful with all these promises because: an excessive emphasis in technological solutions to prevent or treat disease diverts our attention from the root of the problem, bearing in mind that health relies on favourable social circumstances; in addition, clinical medicine and precision prevention have become an industry advertisement tool. Protecting individuals against big corporations in the current political scenario may sound naïve given the constant economic inequalities experienced in the world in the last decades. In a fair world, healthy living directly threatens many powerful corporations.

Overrated precision medicine promises may be serving vested interests, by dictating priorities in the research agenda and justifying the exorbitant healthcare expenditure in our finance-based medicine. If societies aspire to address strong risk factors for non-communicable diseases, they will require downplaying the numerous promises of precision medicine and a greater appreciation of the importance of spending more resources on the foundational conditions that shape the health of the populations (Rey-Lopez, De Sa and De Rezebde, 2018).

In the next coming years, many genomic discovery platforms in combination with clinical phenotyping based on electronic medical record data will lead to more insight with respect to disease processes and lead to more individualised targeted treatment. Overall, the use of clinical phenotype and classification tools help to diagnose disease early to allow a more rapid introduction of targeted treatment avoiding harm and increasing benefit (Twilt, 2016).

It is urgent that global or regional bodies which have the capacity to stimulate development of knowledge through centralised platforms which ensure high quality of qualification and validation of biomarkers get their acts together if we want to make precision medicine a given rather than a fortuitous happening, generating false hope for the patients and the scientific community. Access to patients for clinical research needs new set-ups for rapid identification of patients by sub-groups in a pre-competitive manner for rapid assignment according to target, treatment, and/or trials in the best interest of the patient.

Patients need to be informed about the latest scientific advances, and world also needs a new set-up to ensure high-quality biomarker identification to allow secured treatment access. New solutions are needed for optimal benchmarking of emerging technologies across and within classes of agents. The concept one drug, one target, one protocol; is no longer the way forward. Key questions anticipating the real-life implementation of new drugs need to be addressed early on. Long-term toxicity monitoring of mechanism-based therapies needs a new set-up beyond registration of drugs and into real-life for prolonged time.

Clinical research data sets representing a selection of the population provide robust and systematic longitudinal access to data for learning which must then be confirmed in real-life settings. There is no integrated regional or global solution to optimally learn, across cohorts of patients, patterns of resistance and relapse as patients receive treatments and/or enter clinical trials during the evolution of their disease. This is a major limiting factor in addressing one of the key oncology challenges known as tumour heterogeneity. Integrated solution would be key in addressing regulatory endpoints linked to the current scenario by which the evolution of the disease driven by clonal heterogeneity selection is at stake.

Independent data capture for all types of clinical, biological, and imaging data records alongside biomarker test results and all therapies received, in databases which are constantly curated and annotated, would be critical for benchmarking and validating new clinical trial methodology, as well as benchmarking clinical situations when randomisation may not be possible. Solutions taking the continuum of drug development for optimal access to the forefront clinical trials but that would also enable benchmarking clinical research and real-life could be integrated into new processes, where applied comparative effectiveness research supports the decisions taken by Health Technology Assessment bodies and payers, rather than often too artificially designed registration trials. A major transformation of clinical research building on the strengths and complementarity of stakeholders working alongside new business models must be tackled (Lacombe, Meunier and Golfinopoulos, 2017).

Resource-poor regions will face challenges while adopting artificial intelligence. On one hand, the cost of disruptive technologies might be too high for underdeveloped countries, pushing them further behind in improving healthcare (Mesko, Hetenyi and Gyoffy, 2018). This still stands if it is considered that the use of new technologies could be cost-effective in the long run. On the other hand, underdeveloped countries can be more open to policy changes that would facilitate the adoption of such technologies, which could lead to a more widespread adoption than in developed regions. Examples include how Rwanda opened up its emergency care system to Zipline that produces and operates medical drones across the country (Mesko, Hetenyi and Gyoffy, 2018).

On the level of society, will artificial intelligence shift focus from treatment to prevention? Will artificial intelligence increase the cost of care? Will doctors and medical professionals be more efficient, because artificial intelligence handles some of the time-consuming tasks? Will doctors provide better care in underdeveloped regions with the use of artificial intelligence? And, generally, how will it change the current structures of insurance policies? (Mesko, Hetenyi and Gyoffy, 2018).

References

Bengoechea, J.A. (2012) Infection systems biology: from reactive to proactive (P4) medicine. *Int Microbiol*, 15(2):55-60.

Bronimann, S. et al. (2020) An overview of current and emerging diagnostic, staging and prognostic markers for prostate cancer. *Expert Review of Molecular Diagnostics*, 20(8).

Brothers, K.B. et al. (2019) Reconciling opportunistic and population screening in clinical genomics. *Mayo Clinic Proceedings*, 94 (1), 103-109.

Cornwall, J. et al. (2018) Clinical genomics in physical therapy: where to from here? *Physical Therapy & Rehabilitation Journal*, 98(9), pp. 733-736.

Delaney, S.K. et al. (2016) Toward clinical genomics in everyday medicine: perspectives and recommendations. *Expert Review of Molecular Diagnostics*, 16 (5), 521-532.

Flores, M. et al. (2013) P4 medicine: how systems medicine will transform the healthcare sector and society. *Per Med*, 10(6):565-576.

Fox, S. & Duggan, M. (2013) *Health online*. Washington DC: Pew Internet & American Life Project, p.1.

Garate-Escamila, A.K., El Hassani, A.H. & Andres, E. (2020) Classification models for heart disease prediction using feature selection and PCA. *Informatics in Medicine Unlocked*, 19, 100330.

Ginsburg, G.S. & Phillips, K.A. (2018) Precision medicine: from science to value. *Health Affairs*, 37 (5), 694-701.

Gong, J. et al. (2020) A tool for early prediction of severe coronavirus disease 2019 (COVID-19): a multicentre study using the risk normogram in Wuhan and Guandong, China. *Clinical Infectious Diseases*, 71(15), pp. 833-840.

Hathout, Y. et al. (2016) Clinical utility of serum biomarkers in Duchenne muscular dystrophy. *Clin Proteomics*, 13:9.

Hendriksen J.M.T. et al. (2013) Diagnostic and prognostic prediction models. *Journal of Thrombosis and Haemostasis*, 11(Suppl. 1), pp. 129-141.

Huang, Y. & Zhu, H. (2017) Protein array-based approaches for biomarker discovery in cancer. *Genom Proteom Bioinform*, 15(2), 73-81.

Inoue, Y. et al. (2020) Diagnostic and prognostic biomarkers for chronic fibrosing interstitial lung diseases with a progressive phenotype. *Chest*, 158(2), pp. 646-659.

Iriart, J.A.B (2019) Precision medicine/personalized medicine: a critical analysis of movements in the transformation of biomedicine in the early 21st century. *Cadernos De Saude Publica*, 35(3):e00153118.

ISBUSA (2018) *What is systems biology*. Institute for Health Systems Biology: Seattle.

Jha, M. et al. (2018) Ensemble approach for developing a smart heart disease prediction system using classification algorithms. *Research Reports in Clinical Cardiology*, 9, 33-45.

Johnson, D.S. et al. (2007) Genome-wide mapping of in vivo protein-DNA interactions. *Science*, 16(5830), 1497-1502.

Kalda, R. et al. (2015) *Feasibility study for personalised medicine in Estonia*. University of Tartu.

Khan, M.A. (2020) An IoT framework for heart disease prediction based on MDCNN classifier. *IEEE Access*, 8, pp. 34717-34727.

Lacombe, D. et al. (2017) Precision medicine: from "omics" to economics towards data-driven healthcare – time for European transformation. *Biomedicine Hub*, 2 (suppl 1), 480117.

Long, J.C. et al. (2021) A dynamic systems view of clinical genomics: a rich picture of the landscape in Australia using a complexity science lens. *BMC Medical Genomics*, 63(2021).

Makman, B.T. (2013) *Biomarkers for go/no go decisions*. In: Lenz H-J., editor. Biomarkers in oncology – prediction and prognosis. New York: Springer.

McLellan, S. (2014) Precision medicine: the future of data-driven healthcare. Umea University.

Ministry of Health - Canada (2015) *Unleashing innovation: excellent healthcare for Canada.* Report of the Advisory Panel on Healthcare Innovation. Ottawa.

National Research Council Committee on AFsDaNToD (2011) *Toward precision medicine: building a knowledge network for biomedical research and a new taxonomy of disease.* Washington DC: National Academics Press (US) National Academy of Sciences.

Noble, D. (1960) Cardiac action and pacemaker potentials based on the Hodgkin-Huxley equations. *Nature,* 188:495-497.

Ormondroyd, E. et al. (2018) Not pathogenic until proven otherwise: perspectives of UK clinical genomics professionals toward secondary findings in context of a genomic medicine multidisciplinary team and the 100,000 genomes project. *Genetics in Medicine,* 20 (3), 320-328.

Pellegrini, P. et al. (2011) Gender-specific cytokine pathways, targets, and biomarkers for the switch from health to adenoma and colorectal cancer. *Clin Dev Immunol,* 2011:819724.

Philippi, S. & Kohler, J. (2006) Adrressing the problems with life-science databases for traditional uses and systems biology. *Nat Rev Genet,* 7(6):482.

Pitteri, S. & Hanash, S. (2010) A systems approach to the proteomic identification of novel cancer biomarkers – IOS Press. *Dis Mark,* 28(4).

Primorac, D. et al. (2020) Pharmacogenomics at the center of precision medicine: challenges and perspective in an era of big data. *Pharmacogenomics,* 21(2), pp. 141-156.

Ramaswami, R., Bayer, R. & Galea, S. (2018) Precision medicine from a public health perspective. *Annual Review of Public Health,* 39, pp. 153-168.

Rattan, S. (2018) *Hormones in ageing and longevity.* Springer.

Rey-Lopez, J. et al. (2018) Why precision medicine is not the best route to a healthier world. *Revisa de Saude Publica*, 52:12.

Sagner, M. et al. (2017) The P4 health spectrum – a predictive, preventive, personalised and participatory continuum for promoting healthspan. *Prog Crdiovasc Dis*, 59(5):506-521.

Sandhu, K.V. et al. (2017) Feeding the microbiota-gut-brain axis: diet, microbiome, and neuropsychiatry. *Transl Res*, 179, 223-244.

Sauer, U. et al. (2007) Getting closer to the whole picture. *Science*, 316:550.

Schadt, E.E. et al. (2010) Computational solutions to large-scale data management and analysis. *Nat Rev Genet*, 11(19):647-657.

Sherwin, E. et al. (2016) May the force be with you: the light and dark sides of the microbiota-gut-brain axis in neuropsychiatry. *CNS Drugs*, 30(11), 1019-1041.

Tian, Q. et al. (2017) Systems cancer medicine: towards realization of predictive, preventive, personalized and participatory (P4) medicine. *J. Intern Med*, 271(2):111-121.

Tu, S. et al. (2014) Protein microarrays for studies of drug mechanisms and biomarker discovery in the era of systems biology. *Curr Pharm Des*, 20(1), 49-55.

Twilt, M. (2016) Precision medicine: the new era in medicine. *EBioMedicine*, 4, 24-25.

Vijay, P. et al. (2017) Clinical genomics: challenges and opportunities. *Crit Rev Eukaryot Gene Expr*. 26 (2), 97-113.

Vogt, et al. (2016) The new holism: P4 systems medicine and the medicalization of health and life itself. *Med Health Care Philos*, 19(2):307-323.

Wynants, L. et al. (2021) Prediction models for diagnosis and prognosis of COVID-19: systematic review and critical appraisal. *British Medical Journal* 2020.369m1328.

Don't miss out!

Visit the website below and you can sign up to receive emails whenever Mbuso Mabuza publishes a new book. There's no charge and no obligation.

https://books2read.com/r/B-A-JPJL-PSVKC

BOOKS 2 READ

Connecting independent readers to independent writers.

Did you love *Precision Medicine*? Then you should read *Health Systems Engineering: Building A Better Healthcare Delivery System*[1] by Mbuso Mabuza!

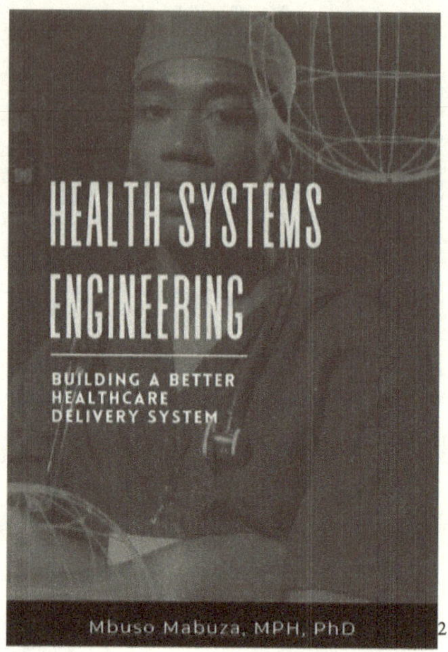

[2]

There is increasing recognition that efforts to improve global health cannot be achieved without stronger health systems.

The myriad of opportunities and challenges that come with rapid technological innovations in the medical and health ecosystem, warrant an urgent need to apply systems engineering techniques and skills to solve issues pertaining to healthcare service quality, patient safety, and healthcare cost, as means to improve healthcare systems performance. Health systems engineering can solve healthcare problems that no one else can.

---

1. https://books2read.com/u/mYQKpo

2. https://books2read.com/u/mYQKpo

Health systems engineering entails the application of engineering, science, management, and technological innovation to healthcare systems improvement. A successful systems engineering delivery process in healthcare should focus on defining stakeholder needs and required functionality early in the development cycle, documenting requirements, then proceeding with design synthesis and system validation while considering the complete problem. It focuses on understanding the interactions among people (patients, families, clinicians, and other stakeholders), processes (institutional, regulatory, professional ethics, etc.), and technology (medical devices and instrumentation) in the healthcare domain to formulate a systems approach to innovations that lead to improved patient outcomes.

The proposed healthcare setting should have the environmental factors desired by patients and family members as expressed by them, suggesting a need for improvements in the healthcare environment. The patient and family must be kept at the centre of the systems approach. There are no technical barriers to enabling that capability, and the payoff in terms of patient and family experience may be substantial.

Perhaps, health is too important to be left only to doctors; the healthcare consumer's well-being should be the primary consideration. The ultimate goal is to ensure that quality goals and objectives of the 21st century health system are achieved through accessible, safe, effective, patient-centred, timely, efficient, and equitable health care.

There is no doubt that very few healthcare professionals or administrators are equipped to think analytically about health care delivery as a system or to appreciate the relevance of systems engineering tool. Even fewer are equipped to work to apply these tools. With the increasing global burden of disease, and the risk of pandemics such as we have already seen with the COVID-19, there is an urgent need to develop and enhance capacity for the design and application of health systems engineering, in order to build a better healthcare delivery system. A very important issue therefore is for the educators, students and practitioners to develop a sound understanding of what health systems engineering actually means. Accordingly, there is a need for multi-skilled professionals with qualifications in health systems engineering.

This book aims to address that need. The book begins with an overview of a systems approach to healthcare. It then discusses health systems including health systems strengthening and the role of knowledge management and leadership, essential health packages, public-private partnerships, healthcare financing, and monitoring performance. Health systems engineering is discussed with a particular focus on engineering better health and care, and on how it can transform the medical and healthcare ecosystem. This book will appeal to professionals and students in medicine and healthcare, global health, public health, health economics, healthcare leadership and management, health systems strengthening and research, healthcare innovations, data analytics and health informatics, systems engineering, sustainable development, public policy, social sciences, and related fields.

Also by Mbuso Mabuza

A Healthy Mind And Best You: Achieving Great Results in Every
Aspect of Your Life
Purposeful And Better You
Sustainable Development Calls for Effective Strategic Leadership for
Efficient Health Systems
Health Promotion In Low Socioeconomic Settings
Medicine and Sociology of Health
Qualitative Methods In Public Health Research
Global Health Disaster Management
Global Health Policy And Programme Challenges
The Journey of Life Has a Gift of Purpose
Epidemiological Research
Ethics, Qualitative And Quantitative Methods In Public Health
Research
When Love Lasts
Blockchain Technology In Healthcare
Virtual and Augmented Reality in Healthcare
Data Analytics and Healthcare Informatics
How To Improve The Way You Think
Health Systems Engineering: Building A Better Healthcare Delivery
System
Artificial Intelligence In Drug Discovery And Development
Precision Medicine

About the Author

Dr Mbuso Mabuza is a highly motivated life-long learner and multi-skilled global health professional. Dr Mabuza's mission is to improve health outcomes and to expand quality healthcare experiences amongst all groups of people and influence change and innovation.